Author

Seongkuk Yoon (Doctor of Korean Medicine)

Bachelor of Korean Medicine of Dong-Shin University in 2003

Certified Korean Doctor passed 59th national qualification
examination of Korean Medicine in 2003

Da-min Korean Medical Clinic in Seoul since 2010

Member of The Society of Korean Medicine

Member of The Association of Korean Medicine

Member of The Society of Internal Korean Medicine

Member of Korean Pharmacopuncture Institute

Member of The Society of Korean Medicine for Obesity Research

Member of The Study of Thread Embedding Acupunture

Table of Contents

Am I overweight?

Normal physical activity requires a lot of energy. All human activities need energy. Even when the body seems to be doing nothing, energy is consumed continuously. That is the basic metabolic rate. The human body continues to work with the heart beating, breathing and maintaining body temperature. For adult men, the basic metabolic rate is about 1600 kcal and for adult women, about 1,100 kcal. In addition to the basic metabolic rate, additional activity consumes more energy. That is active metabolism. The metabolic rate at very light activity is 30% of the basic metabolic rate. And the activity metabolism at extreme exercise is 90% of the basic metabolic rate, but this is temporary. Therefore, if your body has more energy than the body needs for physical activity, you become obese. In that sense, the concept of basic metabolic rate is important for those who want to go on a diet.

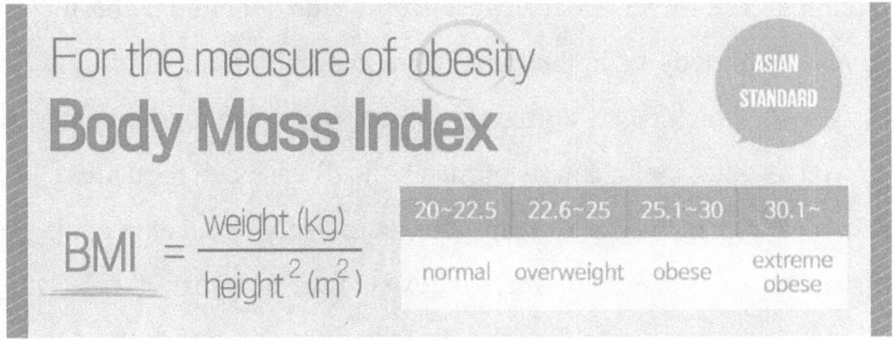

Obesity is a result of a chronic build-up of energy in the form of body fat. However, there are practical difficulties in measuring this professionally. The most accurate measurement of obesity is by CT or MRI, which is a matter of cost and time. There is a measurement with InBody in a simpler way, but this also requires a machine. Since there is a useful method, it is the BMI(body mass index). In reality, it is the most convenient because you can get a body mass index by knowing your weight and height and height. The method by which the body mass index is obtained is by dividing the body weight by the square of the height (kg/m2). The World Health Organization (WHO) divides body mass index 25 to 29.9 into overweight and 30 or higher into obesity. However, it is not suitable for Korean as it is based on the average value of the world. In Asia, including Korea, WTO standards are corrected to treat obesity starting with Body Mass Index 25.

However, BMI also has limitations. This is because each person has different body types. Also, people who exercise a lot or develop muscles naturally can misdiagnose body fat as obesity. In this regard, the most clinically useful indicator is abdominal circumference measurement. Most people with abdominal obesity have a lot of body fat in their gut. More internal fat causes insulin resistance, which increases the risk of diabetes and hyperlipidemia, as well as other major causes of metabolic diseases. In particular, Asian people, including Koreans, are more likely to develop adult diseases even if their body mass index is lower than that of Westerners. However, although CT is the most accurate method to determine the level of abdominal obesity, it is not easy to measure, it is expensive, and there is a risk of radiation exposure. So waist circumference is easily measured in clinical practice. The waist circumference is based on the portion of the boundary below the ribs and the midpoint of the hip bone ridge. For adult males, a waist greater than 90 cm is judged to be abdominal obesity. And for adult women, abdominal obesity is the case with a waist circumference of 85 cm or more.

The true shape of appetite

Humans have been starving since ancient times, and our bodies have evolved to escape hunger. However as times have changed, we are in an unexpected situation. Our bodies are set in the direction of building energy in our bodies, so we don't know how to get rid of obesity. That is why obesity is not something that can be overcome simply by will. In fact, there are many biological factors between hunger and obesity. If you starve, the stomach releases a substance called grelin, which makes you feel hungry. Also, the smell of food, the color and image of food, the memories of eating deliciously, and moods stimulate the dopamine system that causes hunger in our body. For example, there is a rice noodle shop on the way home from work. At first, you are hungry, so you buy and eat rice noodles. So several times you pass by the rice noodle shop. Later, you go and eat rice noodles even if you are not hungry because you are stimulated by the delicious smell of rice noodle shops and pictures of rice noodles. When it is cold or you are depressed, you sometimes eat rice noodles because you remember being happy to have them. The human body's system of getting out of hunger does not stop here. Favorite foods, delicious foods, soft foods to chew easily, high calorie foods, and tasty foods with strong aroma activate the pleasure centers in the brain. When the central nervous system is stimulated like this, you can't stop eating. You eat like a dog.

In fact, the cause of gaining weight is also related to genetics. If parents are fat, chances are about 10 percent that their children will be fat due to genetic effects. There may be a difference between how much food you feel satisfied with your diet, but if you don't feel satisfied relatively well due to genetic effects, you are more likely to become obese. This obesity-related gene mainly affects the level of gastrointestinal movement and hormone secretion. There are also many other factors that are detrimental to people's appetite. First of all, mental stress is increasing. When you are under mental stress, you want to eat high-calorie, high-sugar, and high-fat foods. And this interacts with the stress hormone cortisol, which secrete dopamine, making it eat more food. Next, sleep time also affects obesity. As electricity was invented and sleep time became shorter, the release of the weight-control hormone leptin was reduced, forcing more of the appetite-promoting hormone grelin to be released. In other words, people eat more.

So, is appetite uncontrollable? It's not exactly. If you have the will, you can control your appetite properly. But in order to do so, you have to think slowly first. We habitually think and act on almost everything that is repetitive without much thought. About 90 percent of a person's thoughts and actions are handled by a fast thinking system, and the same is true of eating food. If you don't think consciously when you eat, you will eat a lot according to your past habits. But it doesn't have to do so. And by recognizing that you are eating unconsciously, you can consciously control your appetite. In other words, you should curb your behavior so that you don't eat quickly and impulsively. And you should make a habit of thinking slowly about how much food you will eat. If you create a new habit of treating food this way for a long time, you can control your appetite. Besides that, it's good to exercise. Exercise consumes energy and directly reduces weight, while lowering grelin levels to help control your appetite. Also, increasing sleep time enough helps control your appetite. Because the concentration of leptin, which regulates appetite, is generally adjusted for sleep time, as the concentration of leptin increases between night and dawn, resulting in a decrease in appetite.

The addicted brain makes you obese

Food is not just a means of nutrition. The flavor of the food, the feeling of chewing, the exercise of the chin, and the feeling of satiation after eating are also meaningful. Through these factors, food stimulates the pleasure center of the brain. When the pleasure center is stimulated, you feel better. Some people get rid of their stress when they eat. Eating delicious food changes your mood when you feel bad or depressed. However, the problem is that people can become addicted to pleasure.

Negative emotions or stress, such as depression, are repetitive events. This continues to the moment when a person dies. And then there's someone whose appetite increases. This is the result of learning. If you relieve stress by eating like that, overeating or eating too much is repeated. As this process repeats, the brain can gradually become addicted to food. The obsession with eating food increases, and the desire for food grows. When you are addicted to food, you keep eating even if you are full. The amount of food that you eat increases gradually, so you eat much more often than you used to. When you try to control your food with a firm mind, you may experience withdrawal symptoms such as anxiety, irritation, depression, and headaches. Eating food is more affected by the brain than we think. Some of the major eating disorders that the brain is addicted to food include binge eating disorder and bulimia nervosa.

Binge eating disorder means that binge eating clearly more food in a given amount of time is repeated several times, and that the ability to control what you eat is impaired. What is the clinical significance of binge eating? If you eat more than usual, eat more until you are uncomfortably full, eat a lot of food even though you are not hungry, feel guilty for eating too much, suffer severe stress from binge eating, and binge-eat at least once a week for at least three months, you can be diagnosed with binge eating disorder. Bulimia nervosa is a disease similar to binge eating disorder. Bulimia nervosa is similar to binge eating disorder in that it repeats binge eating, but it is different in that it acts as a reward to avoid weight gain. Typical compensatory behaviors include vomiting after binge eating, abuse of laxatives or diuretics, excessive exercise and fasting. If both binge eating and compensatory behavior show up at least once a week for at least three months, it can be diagnosed with bulimia nervosa. And it is usually seen in young women. It usually begins to appear in adolescence or early adulthood. Antidepressants are usually used in medication for eating disorders, but obesity caused by eating disorders is not simple. There are many causes. We should look at self-esteem, mood swings, frequency of stress, jobs, interpersonal relationships, weight and age. Above all, we must refer to whether they are mentally ill or not.

Other common symptoms include night eating syndrome. Night eating syndrome is the act of waking up or eating food after dinner. They are aware of what they eat on their own and are often stressed out by their eating behavior, which affects their daily lives. Night eating syndrome is highly associated with sleep disorders. Therefore they should try to treat insomnia. In addition, efforts to relieve stress are important to treat night eating syndrome. And stretching to relax muscles is good. Abdominal breathing, which relieves stress and tension, is also effective.

The risk of childhood obesity

Children who gain weight because of eating habits are often taller than their peers. However, if they fail to lose weight and remain obese, chances are high that they will be not only fat but also short when you become an adult. Because of obesity, the growth plate closes early as puberty comes fast. In other words, childhood obesity is not only likely to lead to adult obesity, it also has an adverse effect on height growth. Usually, obesity diagnoses in children and adolescents use body mass index. Comparing body mass index with children of their age, 85th percentile or higher is considered overweight, 95th percentile or higher is considered obese, and 99th percentile or higher is diagnosed with extreme obesity. The body mass index reflects the risk of body fat and obesity complications. So the body mass index is useful because it can be compared with the degree of obesity despite changes in height and weight due to growth.

Why does childhood obesity lead to adult obesity? It's because of fat cells. There is a fixed period of increase in fat cells in the body. Usually, fat cells explode from birth to age 1. After that, fat cells begin to grow around the age of five or six and fat cells increase a lot in adolescence. Especially, if they eat too much high-calorie food at puberty or accumulate nutrients in the body due to lack of activity, the chance of becoming obese increases with the number of fat cells. And the number of fat cells increased during childhood and adolescence lasts a lifetime. Therefore, once the number of fat cells increases due to childhood obesity, it will not only lead to obesity in adults, but it will also lead to weight gain more than others.

And childhood obesity can in itself be a cause of disease. In other words, childhood obesity can cause metabolic syndrome, such as diabetes, hyperlipidemia and high blood pressure, and non-alcoholic fatty liver. Overweight also causes chronic pain in the hip and knee joints, can be cramped in the leg, and can cause deformation in the knee and ankle joints. The circulation to the respiratory tract also worsens, causing snoring, sleep apnea, asthma, and headaches, and in women, it can lead to ovulation caused by polycystic ovarian syndrome. In addition, childhood obesity also causes a lot of stress psychologically, which reduces one's self-esteem. Of course, there are also cases of morbid obesity caused by disease, in addition to simple childhood obesity. Typically, hypothyroidism, growth hormone deficiency and Cushing's syndrome can lead to obesity. In this case, it is necessary to check for underlying conditions and seek treatment, but it does not account for a significant portion of childhood obesity, as it is less than 1 percent of the total.

In fact, most of childhood obesity is a problem for parents. These include genetic factors inherited from parents, but their lifestyles and eating habits are more important than that. According to the survey, even if only one parent is obese, there is a 50 percent chance that their child is obese, and if both parents are obese, there is an 80 percent chance that their child is obese. Parents and children share lifestyle, exercise, food volume, and types of food. And the option is on the parents. Therefore, if parents take the lead, they will reduce the likelihood of obesity in their children.

Skinny fat obesity

There is a BMI (body mass index) as a basic way of determining obesity. Generally, a BMI of 25 or more is judged obese. However, there is obesity that cannot be distinguished by body mass index. It's skinny fat obesity. Skinny fat obesity is an apparently lean body under the normal weight range, but it is a "sarcopenic obesity" that lacks muscle mass in the body. Usually, they have skinny bodies and thin arms and legs, but their lower abdomen is only bulging. Since they are obese due to lack of muscle mass, the proportion of women is higher than that of men. In addition, many elderly people are also seen with reduced muscle mass.

The problem is that skinny fat obesity can be more dangerous than overweight obesity. Because skinny fat obesity with the lack of muscle mass means abdominal obesity with excessive fat accumulation in the gut. Abdominal obesity is the cause of many adult diseases. In other words, abdominal obesity increases blood cholesterol levels and leads insulin resistance. Therefore, the possibility of developing various metabolic diseases such as diabetes, high blood pressure and hyperlipidemia will increase.

So, how do we judge skinny fat obesity? Skinny fat obesity is indistinguishable by body mass index. So, for adults, body fat rates and waist circumference are used, and for older adults, body fat rates and muscle mass are used. Adult men with a body fat ratio of 25% or more and a waist circumference of 90cm or more are judged to be skinny fat obesity. Adult women with a body fat rate of over 30 percent and a waist circumference of over 85 centimeters are judged to be skinny fat obesity. Older men with a body fat rate of 27 percent or more, and those with muscle mass of 7.26kg/m^2 or less are considered to be skinny fat obesity. And an elderly woman with a body fat ratio of 38 percent or more, and a muscle mass of 5.45kg/m^2 or less, is considered to be skinny fat obesity.

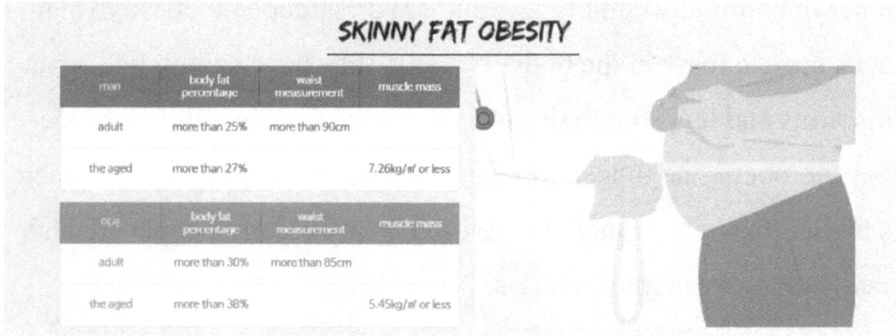

SKINNY FAT OBESITY

man	body fat percentage	waist measurement	muscle mass
adult	more than 25%	more than 90cm	
the aged	more than 27%		7.26kg/㎡ or less

여자	body fat percentage	waist measurement	muscle mass
adult	more than 30%	more than 85cm	
the aged	more than 38%		5.45kg/㎡ or less

There are many causes of skinny fat obesity. For one thing, diet menu is often a problem. In other words, repeated low-calorie diets can significantly reduce muscle mass in the long run, since muscles are first repeatedly decomposed in the early stages. Also, if you enjoy a vegetarian diet, your muscle mass will gradually decrease as your protein intake is likely to be low. Furthermore, if meal times are irregular and binge eating is repeated, the possibility of skinny fat obesity can be even higher because body fat increases sharply. The second problem is lack of exercise. When the amount of exercise is proper, the body fat is decomposed as the muscle mass is maintained. However, a lack of exercise does not reduce body fat and reduces muscle mass. And the body fat fills up as much space as the reduced muscle.

Therefore, it can be dangerous to try to lose too much weight if you are skinny fat. Older adults, in particular, may lose more if they are forced to lose weight. If they go on a low-calorie diet that reduces the amount of food they eat, their skinny fat obesity can worsen, and they can easily lose energy as their muscle mass decreases, which can lead to extreme fatigue. On the other hand, if they rapidly increase their workout, chances of fractures due to osteoporosis are increased. In addition, excessive weight loss can lead to decreased immunity and can often be exacerbated by pneumonia or herpes zoster.

Therefore, if you are skinny fat, you should slowly lose weight in a way that you don't overdo. It is forbidden that eating diets that starve or reduce your diet to an extreme degree. It is important to eat regularly every meal and gradually increase the amount of exercise. First of all, the goal is to maintain your current weight. You should also take calcium and vitamin D in moderation so that you can get enough protein and not weaken your bones. In addition, if you exercise, it is effective to perform low-intensity muscle exercises rather than aerobic exercises.

Diet menu

Dietary controls are essential for successful weight loss. Making a good diet and doing it properly is 80% of the weight loss success. here are many different kinds of weight-loss diets on the market. There are many diets that limit the amount of food you eat, and there are many one-food diets that only consume one kind of food. Of course, you will lose weight at first, but from a long-term perspective, you should be careful because it can cause health problems. In order to lose weight in good health, you must first be able to calculate the right calories for you. And it is advisable to consume a little less calories than the usual energy needs. Proper calories for weight loss can be set to reflect weight, obesity, activity, age and gender. If you take 500 kcal less than you normally need for diet, you can lose 0.5 to 1 kg per week. And if you take 1000 kcal less, you can lose 1 to 2 kg per week. It is desirable to reduce the weight by 500 to 1,000 kcal in order to continue to the extent that it does not harm your health. And beyond that, extreme low-calorie diets can cause many side effects as well as difficulty in continuing your diet.

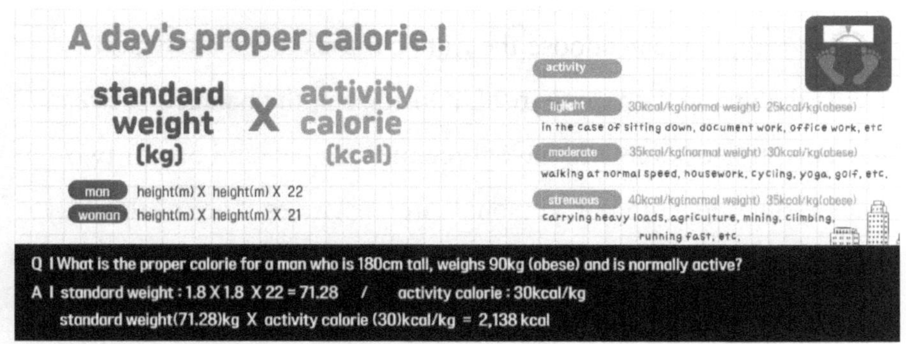

proper calorie count

In a weight-loss diet, there is more to consider in addition to proper calories. That is, balance between nutrients such as carbohydrates, fats, proteins and minerals. This requires proper consumption of grains, meat, fish, eggs, beans, vegetables, fats, dairy products and fruits. The grains such as rice, rice cake, corn, and sweet potatoes contain mainly carbohydrates. Meat, fish, eggs, beans, tofu and nuts are mainly rich in protein. Vegetables and seaweed are rich in vitamins, minerals, and fiber. Sesame oil, wild oil, olive oil, and butter contain a lot of fat. Dairy products such as milk, yogurt and cheese are high in protein and minerals. Also, various fruits contain not only vitamins and minerals, but also carbohydrates.

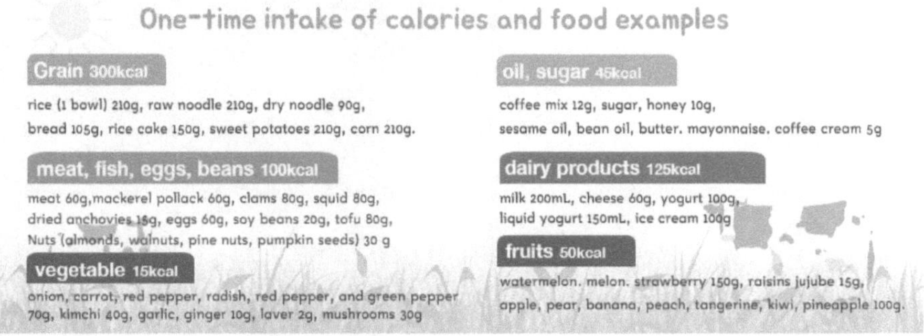

a single-take calorie

In this way, you can choose the right calories to eat a day and decide the diet to eat in one meal, considering the balance between nutrients. It is desirable to have three meals a day and one or two snacks. But depending on personal circumstances, two meals a day and one or two snacks may be made up. Also, for two meals a day, one can eat breakfast and lunch and starve for dinner. It is also possible to eat lunch and dinner and starve breakfast. Eating two meals a day is more effective for diets, as it increases the amount of time you burn fat from your body due to a drop in blood sugar.

Obesity is associated with several metabolic disorders and chronic degenerative diseases. To reduce the risk of getting various adult diseases due to obesity and to maintain a healthy life, one must reduce one's weight to an appropriate level. To this end, a balanced diet between nutrients is essential, reducing intake calories. Repeating ultra-low-calorie diets or following the trend of one-food diets increases the risk of losing weight and becoming obese due to yo-yo.

Exercise for weight loss

Exercise is an effective supplement to losing weight and an important preventative way to keep your weight down. There have been several studies on the effects of exercise on weight. According to a number of papers, a steady stream of exercise, which required endurance without limiting food, resulted in an average weight loss of 3 kilograms for men and an average 1.4 kilograms for women. Exercise-induced diet effects are more pronounced in men than in women, but continuous exercise also has a distinct effect in women. Any exercise may have the effect of losing weight, but for a more efficient weight loss, aerobic exercise and muscular exercise should be used in a proper combination.

Aerobic exercise is a full-body exercise that uses up fat and carbohydrates by supplying oxygen during exercise. Aerobic exercise is more weight-loss effective than muscular exercise because it can burn more fat efficiently. Types of aerobic exercise include walking, running, biking, jumping rope, climbing stairs, swimming, aerobics and badminton. On the other hand, muscular exercise, which increases muscle volume by contracting muscles, has no greater weight loss effect than aerobic exercise. However, muscular exercise can raise the basic metabolic rate because it increases the muscle mass that is reduced by dieting. Continuing a diet reduces muscle mass and reduces basal metabolic rate, which leads to a period of stagnation that does not lose weight well. You can improve your diet's efficiency if you carry out proper muscular exercises. Also, if you enforce muscular exercise well, you can recover figure from repeated diet failures. Therefore, for a successful diet, it is recommended to implement muscular exercise at the same time, based on aerobic exercise, which is good for weight loss.

However, you should not exercise too much in advance of your motivation from the beginning of your diet. In the early part of the diet, weight loss through diet control should be the basis, and exercise should begin slowly with the lowest intensity of exercise. Exercise is more important in frequency and duration than strength. It is recommended to exercise four to five days a week for the first time and 30 to 60 minutes a day. If someone hasn't exercised at all, don't overdo it, start with 10 minutes, three times a week, and slowly expand with his body. In particular, it is recommended to start with less strain on the joints, such as walking, swimming, walking in water, and biking, as the stress on the knees and ankles can be put on when a person starts exercising. Jogging is not recommended because it puts a lot of strain on the knees and joints.

In fact, just increasing physical activity in daily life, as well as exercising, becomes an exercise for weight loss. It is also good to reduce one's computer time and make a habit of walking short distances. It is also possible to use public transportation as usual, and to park cars far away from his destination to increase one's walking distance. And it is a good idea to measure and manage one's physical activity with a pedometer to find out how long he walked a day. Exercise can be a very effective way to diet, but excessive exercise can be a reason for harming your health and stopping your diet. When you exercise to lose weight, it is important to set your target weight, check your body condition, and exercise accordingly.

Maintaining the lost weight

Dieting can be divided into managing weight gain, actively losing weight, and maintaining lost weight. And anyone with diet experience knows that it is more difficult to maintain a reduced weight than to lose weight. It takes more than twice as long to invest in maintaining lost weight than in losing weight. In addition, the yoyo phenomenon of gaining weight again is very common. There are many factors here. Among other things, the problem is the reduced amount of muscle in the diet process. A decrease in muscle mass also reduces the basic metabolic rate. If your basic metabolic rate decreases, you gain weight by increasing body fat even if you eat a little. And the more you go on a diet, the faster and stronger the yo-yo is because your body adapts to your attempt to lose weight. Therefore, in order to maintain a weight loss, an approach that is different from a weight-loss diet is needed.

In fact, the effort to maintain weight should last a lifetime. In particular, to maintain a successful weight, intensive care is needed for the initial six months to one year. The human body tends to maintain homeostasis to the internal environment. A person tends to keep a person's weight constant, just as his or her body temperature always stays constant. So if you don't try to maintain your weight loss, you tend to go back to your weight before you go on a diet. Therefore, it is very important to manage your body to adapt to your new weight.

So, what is the most important thing to maintain lost weight? It's exercise. The most necessary thing to maintain lost weight is exercise. In order to do so, it is better to do sports that are usually interesting than sports that are unfamiliar or boring. This is because they need to increase their muscle strength. It is best to exercise steadily. In addition, it is better to exercise with multiple people or with support from others than to exercise alone. If you are busy or have no time to exercise for personal reasons, you may plan to increase your daily activities sufficiently. For example, it would be a good idea to set a daily walking goal and plan a movement to fill the target until you get home, or to have a habit of using public transportation when commuting.

And diet menu is important in keeping weight, along with exercise. First, it is important to eat three meals a day regularly. In particular, it is recommended that breakfast is not skipped, and three meals a day be distributed evenly. Sometimes social life can only lead to binge-eating or binge drinking, and at this time, you don't have to blame yourself too much. One meal a week does not change your weight easily when you enter the weight retention period. Rather, it is necessary to be flexible in dealing with the situation so as not to be too desperate at this time.

In fact, going on a diet is not an easy task. It takes at least three months to a year to reach weight retention. It's a pain to put up with what you want to eat during this period. Depending on their preferences, many people suffer from stress, anxiety and depression. Psychological problems should not be overlooked in order to wrestle with weight for a long time. Therefore, when there is a disturbance of emotions, it is important to tell the people around you honestly about your state of mind to get encouragement and help.

The Types of diet pills prescribed by doctors

The key to diet is to limit proper calorie intake and increase physical activity. However, if there are difficulties in implementing these factors, medication can be used at the same time. The drugs used in diet can be divided into drugs that reduce calorie intake and those that increase energy consumption. Some of the leading drugs prescribed are Xenical, Belviq, Qsymia, Contrave and Saxenda.

Xenical

Xenical reduces weight by excreting about 30 percent of the fat in the digestive system without absorbing it. As a result, cholesterol, blood pressure and blood sugar levels can be lowered, but HDL-cholesterol levels, which are good cholesterols, can also be reduced. The side effects of Xenical usually appear in the digestive tract. Typically, there are steatorrhea, fecal incontinence, and defecation discomfort.

Belviq

Belviq acts selectively on areas related to appetite among serotonin receptors in the hypothalamus, suppressing appetite and increasing early satiety. Side effects of Belviq include headaches, dizziness, dry mouth and constipation. Currently, Belviq can be prescribed to obese patients with diabetes, obese patients with high blood pressure, severe snoring, reflux esophagus and non-alcoholic fatty liver, obese patients with depression, and obese patients with osteoarthritis.

Qsymia

Qsymia is a drug that mixes the appetite suppressant Phantomine with Topiramate, a treatment for cerebral infarction. Qsymia has increased weight loss effects while halving the capacity of the previously prescribed Phantomine, and the topiramate included in Qsymia has the effect of making patients feel satisfied after meals. Qsymia can be prescribed for the purpose of weight loss to patients with metabolic diseases such as type 2 diabetes, high blood pressure and high cholesterol. However, Qsymia is reported to have an increased risk of developing fetal deformities, so it is safe to check for pregnancy before taking them and to perform contraception during the period of use.

Contrave

Contrave is a drug that combines Naltrexon, which is used in the treatment of alcoholism, with a non-smoking aid called Boupropion. Contrave worked particularly well for people who ate heavily. Side effects of Contrave include nausea, constipation, headaches, vomiting, dizziness, insomnia and diarrhea.

Saxenda

Saxenda is a drug that only differs in name and capacity from Victoza, which is used as a treatment for diabetes, and reduces weight by reducing appetite. There may be nausea, vomiting and diarrhea between the first one or two weeks of the dose, but if taken continuously, side effects tend to decrease gradually.

Disease-induced obesity

Getting fat doesn't end up as just a matter of body figure. Obesity is directly linked to many diseases. Diabetes is the most well-known cause of obesity. The incidence of type 2 diabetes tends to increase from the Body Mass Index of 25, which is also the criterion for judging obesity. In addition, many reports say that for normal people whose body mass index exceeds 30 - the standard for extreme obesity - the death rate from cardiovascular disease increases. Studies show that obese people suffering from diabetes or cardiovascular disease can significantly normalize their blood sugar and blood pressure even if they reduce their weight by five to 10 percent. And there are numerous other diseases that can be caused by obesity. Examples include cataracts, strokes, cognitive impairment, sleep apnea, high blood pressure, hyperlipidemia, liver disease, gallbladder disease, cancer, menstrual impotence, infertility, polycystic ovarian syndrome, arthritis and gout.

Among them, infertility is serious. Obesity works against pregnancy. Obesity has a deep relationship with anovulation. If polycystic ovary syndrome is added to this, its effects are doubled. Polycystic ovary syndrome is a syndrome in which many small cysts are formed in the ovary due to hormonal imbalance, with enlarged ovaries and various special symptoms. It is found in 5-10% of women in the term of pregnancy, and obesity is observed in 35% to 40% of polycystic ovary syndrome. And menstrual disorders and hypertrichosis are more apparent in obese women with polycystic ovary syndrome than normal-weight women with polycystic ovary syndrome. Obesity, in other words, adversely affects women's ovulation and pregnancy through many complex channels. In addition, the more obese women are, the more likely they are to develop polycystic ovary syndrome, and if the two factors appear together, they are more likely to become infertile. And obesity affects the fetus as well. An obese mother's fetus is more likely to have a large baby and congenital malformation, which increases her chances of having a hard time giving birth. Also, newborn babies born to obese mothers are at a higher risk of being overweight at 12 weeks of age compared to those of normal mothers. It appears that environmental and genetic factors work together.

  Conversely, the disease can cause people to get fat. Endocrine diseases such as Cushing's syndrome and growth hormone deficiency are typical. Cushing's syndrome is an endocrine disease in which blood cortisol concentrations are chronically excessive due to a number of causes, such as pituitary adenoma, adrenal hyperplasia, adrenal tumor, and ectopic ACTH secretion. Cushing's syndrome results in weight gain, with the abdomen becoming obese, but the limbs tapering off. In addition, there are more body hair, bruises, and chapped flesh in the abdomen. In the case of growth hormone deficiency, abdominal obesity is also present with significant short stature. Or drugs can cause obesity. It is a case of gaining weight as a side effect of drugs. Some of the drugs that can cause obesity include tricyclic antidepressant, psychotropic substances, steroids, and

Sulfonylurea. If you are good at sports and diet, but you don't lose weight, you should suspect that you are obese due to drugs. And if the drug turns out to be a problem, it will have to be replaced with another set of drugs.

Title : Diet Guide

Subtitle : the essential guide for weight loss

Author : Seongkuk Yoon (DKM)

Publishing company : HealingLife books

Publishing date : 2019.05.20

E-mali : yoonpd3326@gmail.com

ISBN : 9791196474072